AF412851

Handbook
of Clinical
Dermatoglyphs

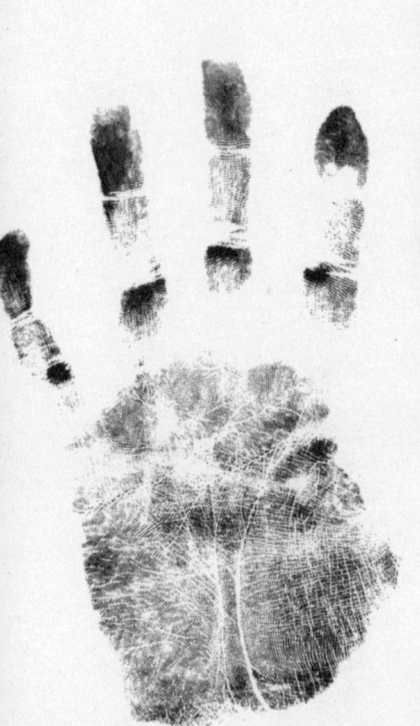

Handbook of Clinical Dermatoglyphs

By

Musallam S. Elbualy and
Joan D. Schindeler

University of Miami Press
Coral Gables, Florida

Contents

Preface

There have been several books written on dermatoglyphics (see bibliography). In general these books are too complex for someone not expert in this subject. It is our feeling that, because of too much detail and complex illustrations, these texts tend to frighten those novices that attempt to use them. On the other hand, there have appeared a number of articles on the subject in various medical journals. In contrast to the textbooks, the articles are not comprehensive; also they are often wordy and not well illustrated.

Because of the increasing usefulness of dermatoglyphics in clinical medicine and the lack of a suitable text, the authors decided to put together this handbook. The subject has been simplified greatly, and illustrations have been used freely with only annotations rather than long descriptions. In this way, it is hoped, the user will be able to compare quickly and easily the findings on his patient with the handbook.

This book is intended for the use of physicians who are not expert in this field and for house staff and other persons in the medical field. A bibliography is provided for those readers who may want to explore the field further. We also hope that some readers (for example physicians in private practice) may be stimulated to set up their own research studies in dermatoglyphics.

Musallam S. Elbualy
Joan D. Schindeler

University of Miami
Mailman Center for Child Development

Introduction

History and Uses of Dermatoglyphs

The study of dermatoglyphics, a name coined by anatomist Harold Cummins in 1926, can trace its beginnings to the late seventeenth century and a physician named Nehemiah Grew. With Dr. Grew's description of the "innumerable little ridges of equal bigness," there were no notable advances until the nineteenth century.

Frances Galton, a cousin of Charles Darwin, set up the first scientific classification of finger skin patterns in 1892. This method is still in use. Skin patterns are produced by a system of parallel lines called ridges with depressions between them known as furrows. The formation of ridges begins early in fetal life, and by eighteen to twenty weeks they are completely formed. Once formed, the patterns are permanent but enlarge with body growth.

In 1936 Cummins published his work on the dermatoglyphic findings in mongol children. In 1959 it was discovered that mongols had a chromosomal abnormality. The association of abnormal chromosomes and dermatoglyphics in the mongol led investigators to look at the association between dermatoglyphics and other conditions with and without abnormal chromosomes. Since then a number of conditions have been found to show ridge pattern combinations that are characteristic. It must be pointed out that not all the patients with a syndrome will individually show the classical ridge patterns known to occur in the syndrome. Not all patients with a disease individually have all the signs and symptoms of that disease either. In the text, classic dermal ridge findings are presented, and whenever possible some variants. Dermatoglyphic formation is under the control of many genes. Therefore, unless exactly the same genes were affected and in the same way, patients with the same syndrome would not show the same dermatoglyphic pattern. Environmental factors can also affect ridge formation in utero.

The use of dermatoglyphics in clinical medicine is facilitated by the fact that the patterns are easily available for study. They can be observed and recorded easily and study is nontraumatic to the patient. The handbook will illustrate conditions where the dermatoglyphs are well defined and will also mention the indefinite findings in other conditions. Dermatoglyphics may also be used to help diagnose zygosity of twins—in monozygotic twins the main characteristics are similar whereas in the dizygotic the dermatoglyphics are no more similar than in other siblings. Dermatoglyphics may suggest a diagnosis when the other manifestations of a condition are not apparent. There are two problems in the clinical use of dermatoglyphics: one is that often in the newborn the ridges are poorly formed and it may be difficult to see the pattern, especially in the premature baby; the other problem is that the person using this diagnostic tool may expect more from it than it can provide. As with any diagnostic tool if it is used in conjunction with other findings, it can indeed help build a case for a particular diagnosis.

Dermatoglyphs, strictly speaking, do not include the flexion crease of palms, soles, and digits. However, mention is usually made of these, e.g., the simian line. This line occurs normally and in many syndromes. Unfortunately, the simian line has become well known to individuals who have little other knowledge of dermatoglyphics, and some of them believe that it is pathognomonic of Down's syndrome (mongolism). Thus, many children especially in the newborn period have been labeled Down's syndrome because they had a simian line. The simian line does occur in Down's syndrome, but there are several ridge patterns that are more diagnostic. The simian line alone without dermatoglyphic findings and without clinical features is not diagnostic of Down's syndrome. The authors hope that the diagnostic faith in the simian line with regard to Down's syndrome will be dispelled.

Techniques in Dermatoglyphs

Man has been recording dermatoglyphs since time aboriginal, and the interest still persists.

The ridges may be viewed by the naked eye with the proper light angle provided they are large and well developed. This is so in adults and children beyond the first months of life. Often a 2.5X magnifying glass is helpful.

When observing the palms and soles, the fingers and toes should be pointing in an upward direction. This position facilitates identification of the pattern types since all graphic illustrations of dermatoglyphs are presented in this way.

Viewing dermal ridges of newborns can seldom be accomplished with the naked eye. We have found that a "flash magnifier" used by stamp collectors is most helpful. This is a small 5X magnifying glass attached to a flashlight base, holding two size C batteries and a light bulb. The illumination is particularly helpful. Another advantage to this flash magnifier is its size. The overall length is only seven inches and will fit easily in a coat pocket. We use the "Selsi flash magnifier," which is made in Japan and sells for approximately two dollars. Naked eye or magnified observation of the patterns is enough for diagnostic purposes. If one wants to have a record of the pattern, prints may be taken.

The techniques for taking good prints vary with the type of ink used. There are three types of ink in the most common usage. The Searche Company manufactures an ink in use by most police departments. This is an undesirable method for our purposes because it blackens the skin and generally is too difficult to control. The advantage of this ink is its permanence.

The ink most popular in the field of dermatoglyphs is manufactured by Faurot, Inc. This is a clear liquid used with an applicator. The special paper is sensitized to the ink and leaves the hand only slightly sticky. These prints fade in about four to five years.

Another fine printing material is made by Hollister of Chicago. This is a dry printer which when used with their glossy paper produces an excellent print. Hollister also produces a Disposable Footprinter, which gives a very black print with well defined ridges. Both these printers are used for palms and soles.

In the newborn the palms and soles should be wiped with an alcohol sponge before applying the ink. This removes any vernix, blanket fuzz, or dead skin. Using the Hollister dry printer, rub gently along the hallucal area of the foot, holding the toes back. When using the Hollister Disposable Foot-printer merely touch the plate to the part that is to be printed. Without too much pressure, roll the glossy side of the paper from the tibial border to the fibular border so as not to miss any triradii. You will find that the Hollister dry printer will need to be scraped with a single edge razor blade from time to time to remove grease from the skin. Sometimes heating the plate in front of a space heater will facilitate the printing.

One should ink the entire hand and attempt to print it, if only to illustrate the overall size and shape of the hand. It is rare that all digital and palmar triradii can be printed at one time. Reink just the palmar area. Be certain to cover the triradius under each digit (the interdigital area). Press gently with the paper. This process may need repeating to assure that all triradii are present on one print. Next, ink each digit and roll the paper across the fingertip to print, remembering to label them thumb, 1, then 2, 3, 4, and 5.

It should be remembered that obtaining readable prints of newborns is a time consuming job and cannot be rushed.

When printing older children and adults the process is basically the same, though simplified.

The Faurot method, because of its cleanliness, is the most popular method and comprises an applicator, ink, and sensitized paper. With an eye dropper apply the ink to the applicator until it is damp. This will probably last through three or four printings. Ink the hand, being certain not to miss the interdigital and lower palm areas.

Place the paper, glossy side up, on a thin piece of foam rubber; hold hand as shown in photo 1. For the best printing, hold the paper with the foam rubber flat on your right palm. Place the patient's hand in the center of the paper. Press the fingers of your right hand into the palm of the patient to obtain a complete palm print (see photo 2). Print the fingertips separately, remembering to number them.

The sole and toes are inked the same way as the palms. The toes will need to be printed separately. They should be held back with the right hand while the paper is pressed

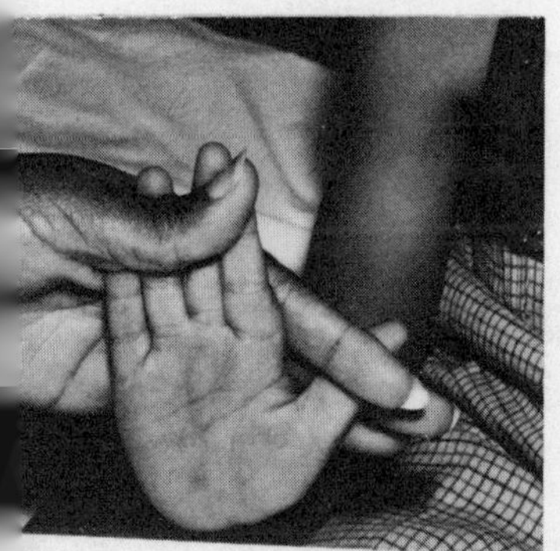

1

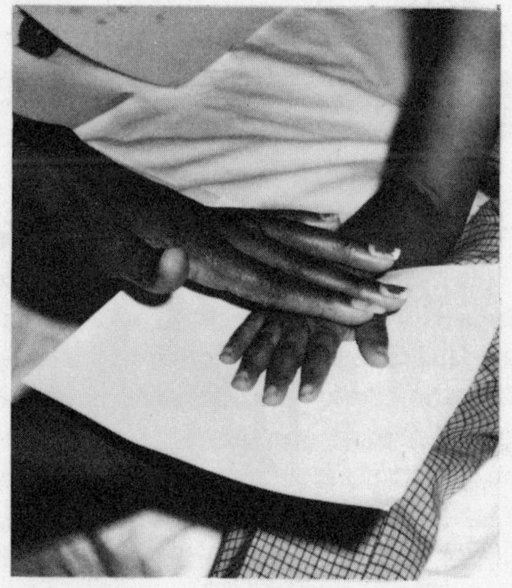

2

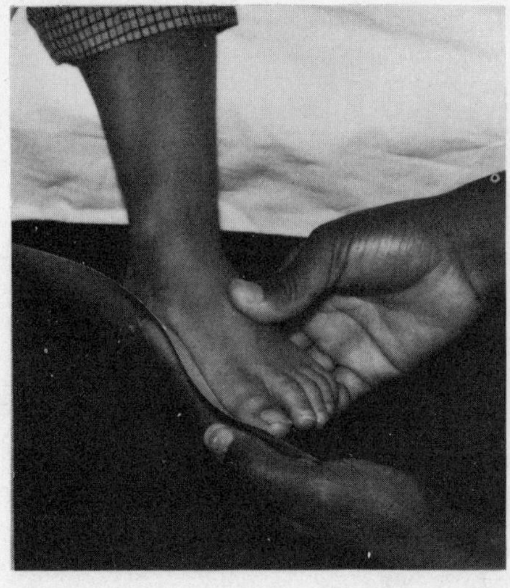

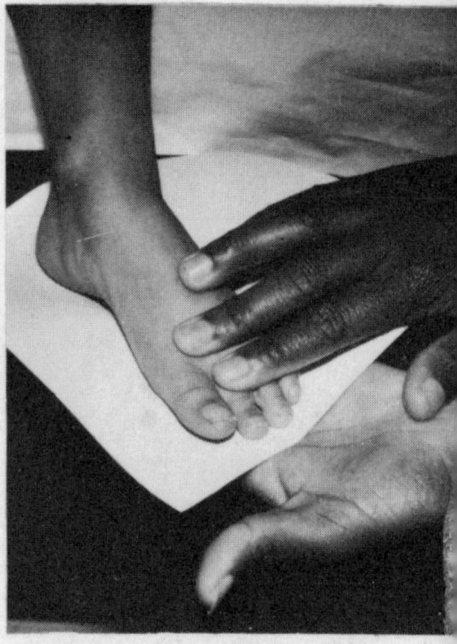

3   4

under them, then up (see photo 3). The reason being the triradii lie close to the crease in the underside of the toe.

The most important area of the sole is the hallucal area. Remember to roll the paper starting up on the tibial side (see photos 3 and 4). The *f* triradius oftentimes lies far up on this border.

When readable prints have been taken, the classifications may vary from a very simple one, which will be presented here, to classifications that have been computerized.

Sometimes it is impossible to get prints, as in the case of a premie in an incubator, hypoplasia, extremely dry skin, etc. By using hand and foot outlines (see Appendix A), one can draw in the type of print as you view it with a magnifying glass or flash magnifier.

Classification of Dermatoglyphs

An international classification of ridge patterns was established in September 1967 in London, England. To understand dermatoglyphic classification one must familarize oneself with the most important term used in the classification, "triradius." The triradius is the center, or junction, of three streams of ridges. This is the point at which all classifications begin (see page 22).

There are five basic digit patterns on the hand (see pages 21 and 22): the arch with no triradii, the loop (either ulnar or radial), with one triradius, and the whorl and the double loop, each with two triradii. Generally, for research purposes the whorls and double loops are reported under one classification, that of whorl. Numerous other "accidental" patterns occur but to keep this text simple these will not be described.

The palm is divided into three large areas: (1) the interdigital area, which lies below and in between digits; (2) the thenar area; and (3) the hypothenar area (see page 24).

There is a triradius at the base of each digit with the exception of the thumb. Starting with the index finger, this triradius is labeled the *a* triradius, the third finger triradius is called the *b*, next the *c*, and then the *d* (see page 24). Occasionally there is a second triradius; this is classified with a prime mark and the letter from the triradius it lies close to, for example *a'*, *b'*, etc. Of the three sets of intersecting ridges that make up a triradius, the line which leaves the triradius area and travels across or down the palm carries the letter designated for the triradius where it began. The "main line," as it is called, is labeled with a capital letter: A, B, C, D. The main lines run in a horizontal direction on the palm (see page 25).

The area between digital triradii is called interdigital: I, between the thumb and index finger; II, between the second and third digit; III, between the third and fourth digit; and IV, between the fourth and fifth digits (see page 24). The most common pattern in these areas is a small loop opening in a distal direction. Whorls are rare.

An *ab* ridge count may be called for in some instances, i.e., Turner's syndrome, Klinefelter's syndrome. This count is a good index of pattern intensity and is independent of age (see page 24). The same rules for doing digital ridge counts apply here. One counts in a straight line from triradius *a* to *b*, including any ridge which the line crosses. The count is reported as summed for both hands. The normal as reported by Pons is: Male 82, Female 84.

The thenar area lies at the base of the thumb. The ridge patterns of this area are classified as loop or positive. The pattern, when it is not a loop, tends to become very complex in this area, and therefore no classification name, letter, or numeral has been given to it by the international group.

The hypothenar area lies on the ulnar portion of the palm extending into the center. There are four primary types of ridge patterns in this area: whorls, loops, arches, and S patterns. Another important triradius occurs in the hypothenar area at the base of the palm. This is called the *t* triradius (axial triradius). Its position on the palm is of important clinical significance (see page 23). By drawing a line from the *a* and *d* triradius to the *t* triradius, the *atd* angle is obtained (see page 23). The angle is measured by protractor. When there is an *a* plus *a'* triradius the most lateral *a* is used, and in the case of the *d* triradius the most medial *d* is used. The *t* may move in a distal direction into the center of the palm; when this occurs another triradius usually is present at the base of the palm. Three positions have been designated for the *t* triradius with corresponding angles: $t = 45^O$, $t' = 51^O$, and $t'' = 56^O$ and over (see page 24). The most distal *t* is always used for the *atd* angle. The position of this distal *t* will give an estimate of the *atd* angle without having to draw it.

The *atd* angle has proved to be a most useful measurement for normal and abnormal palm patterns. The angle does change with palmar growth, but it is sufficient to use a value of 45° as a normal *atd* angle. An angle less than 45° is also normal.

The patterns on the toes are basically the same as on the fingers. The arch with no triradius, the loop (either tibial or fibular) with one triradius, and the whorl and double loop, each with two triradii. There is a triradius at the base of each toe (see page 27). Under the large toe it is designated as *e*, second toe *a*, third *b*, fourth *c*, and fifth *d*. There is a triradius on the tibial border called *f*, and one in the center of the foot called *p*.

The interdigital areas fall between the digital areas as on the palm: the first, between the large and second toe; the second, between the second and third toe; the third, between third and fourth toes; and the fourth, between fourth and fifth toes.

Classification of the entire sole is both complex and unagreed upon. The sole has one area that will be classified in this text. This is the large area under the big toe and lying on the tibial border. It is called the hallucal area. Patterns in this area resemble hypothenar patterns.

3

Normal Dermatoglyphs

TYPES OF DIGITAL PRINTS

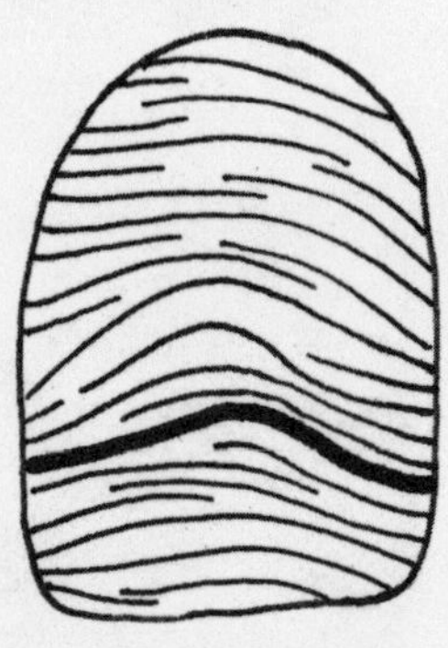

Arch

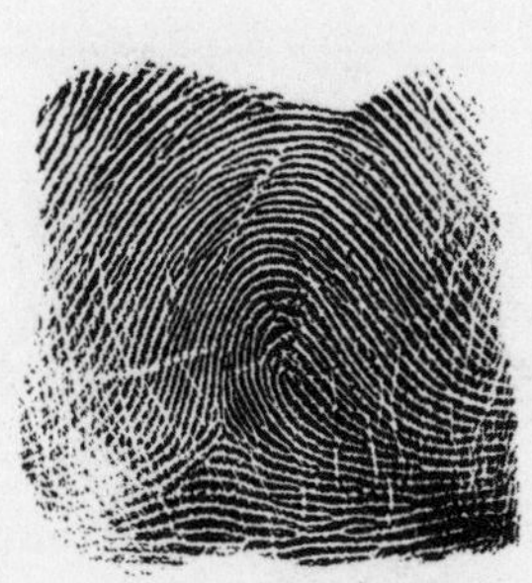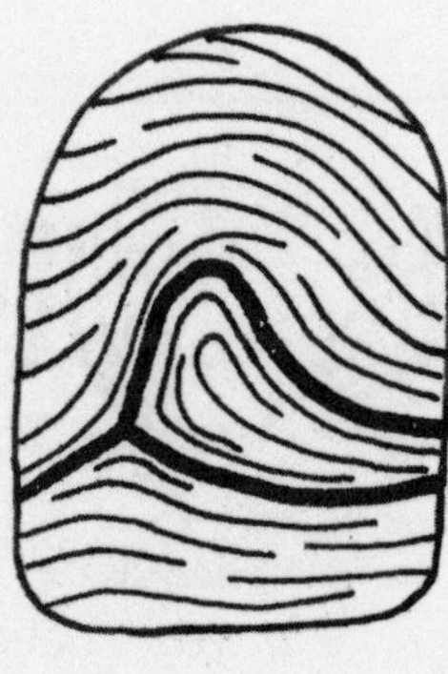

Loop

TYPES OF DIGITAL PRINTS (Continued)

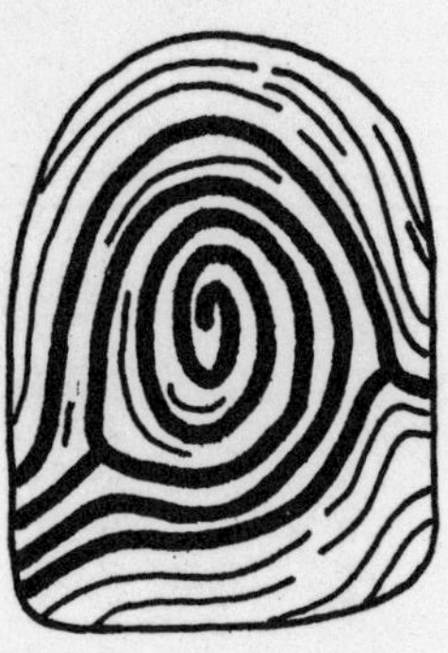

Whorl

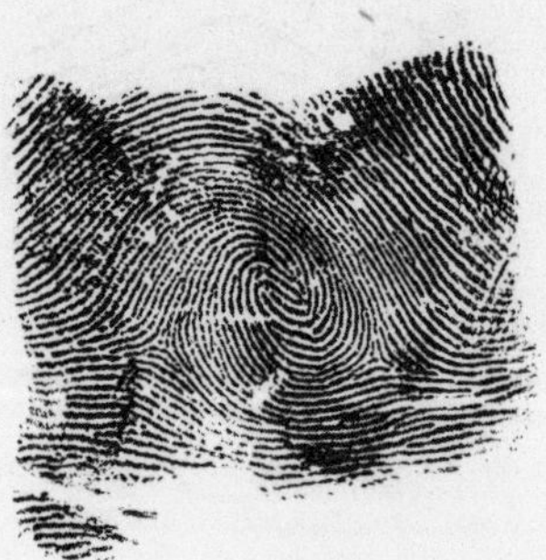
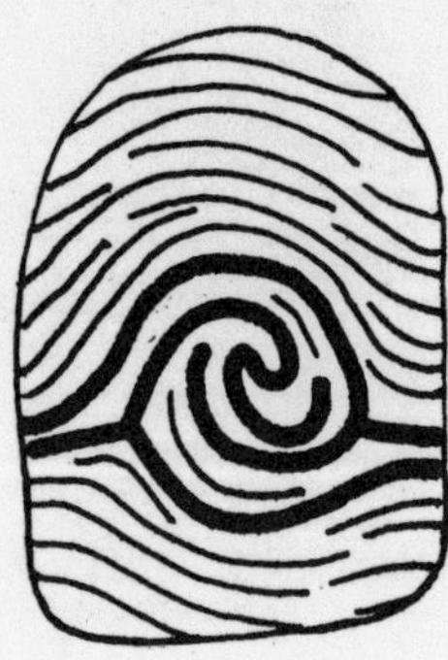

Double loop

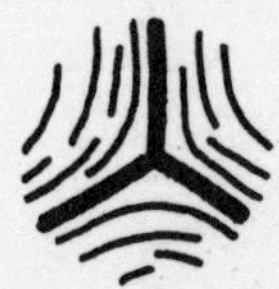
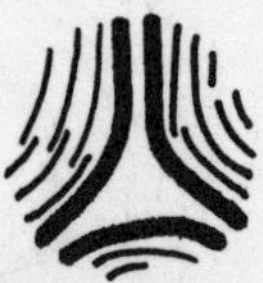
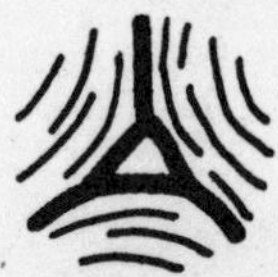

Triradius - The center, or junction, of three streams of ridges. Four examples of triradii. Note that in some cases it is an arbitrary point.

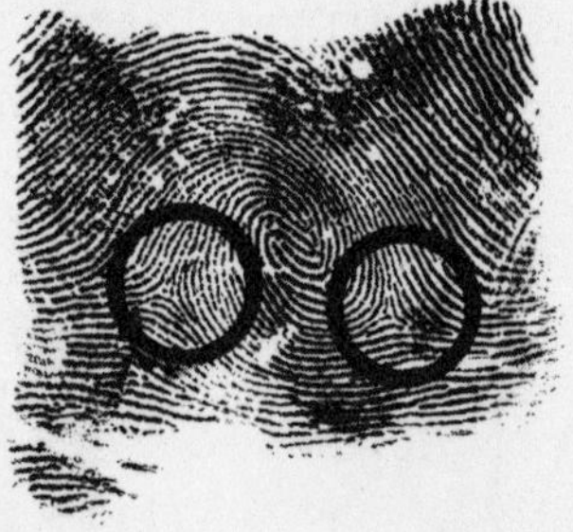

Double loop with two triradii

atd ANGLE

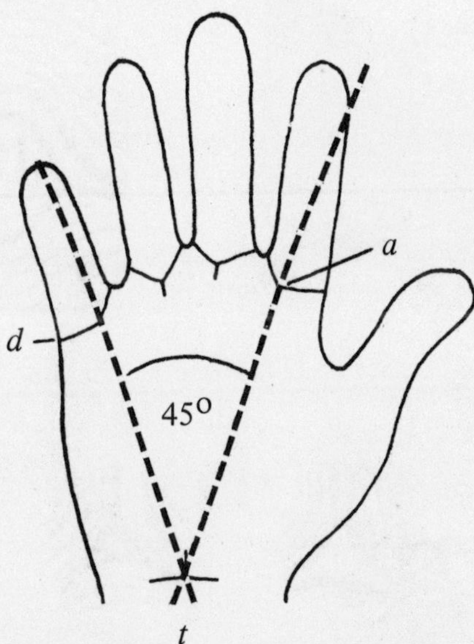

atd Angle - *atd* angle subtended by lines drawn from the *t* triradius to the *a* and *d* triradii.

CLASSIFICATION OF HAND PRINT

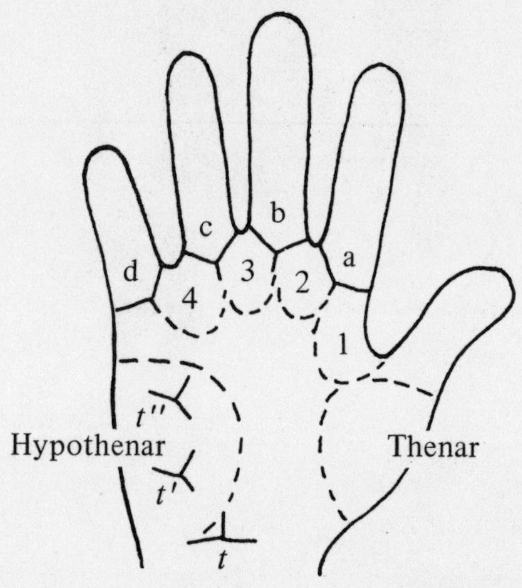

1, 2, 3, 4 = Interdigital areas
a, b, c, d = Digital triradii
t, t', t'' = Axial triradii

EXAMPLE OF AN *AB* RIDGE COUNT

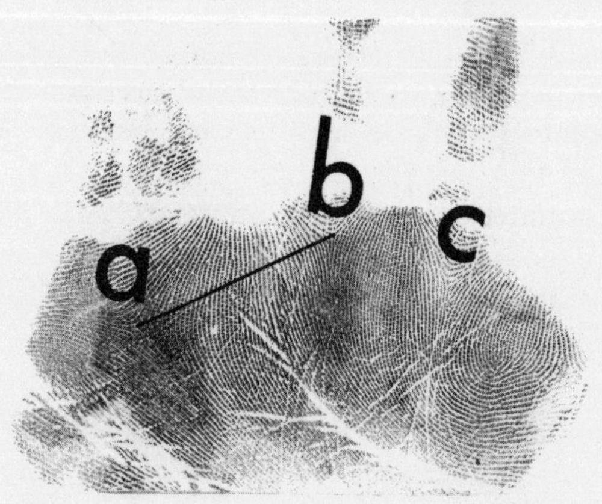

CLASSIFICATION OF MAIN LINES

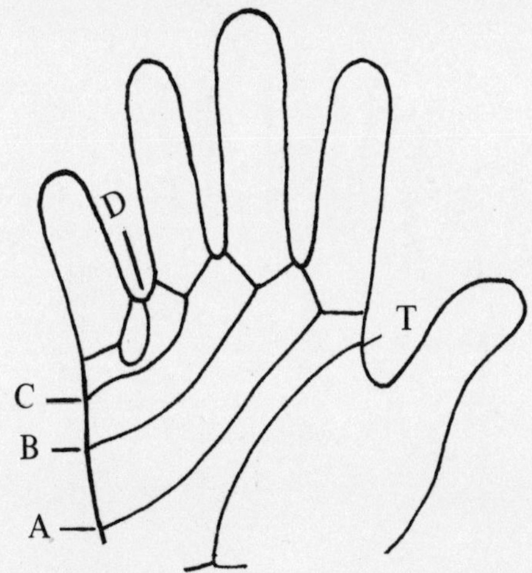

RIDGE COUNTING

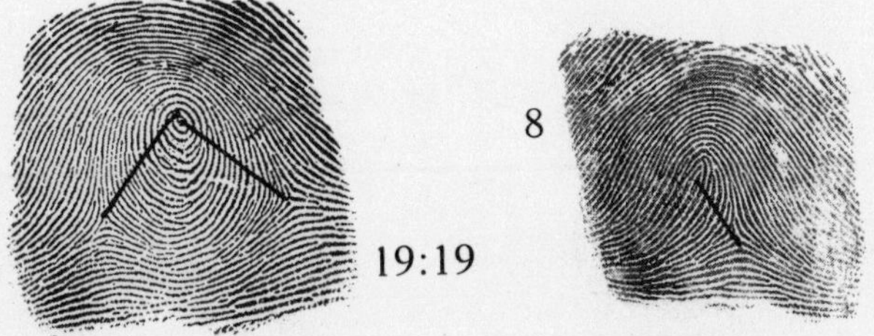

The ridge count is done under low magnification. The ridge count consists of the number of ridges between the triradius and the point of core, or center of the pattern. Neither the triradius nor the final ridge when it forms the center of the pattern is counted. In the case of whorl, both sides of the pattern are counted (see above) and the higher count is reported for a total ridge count. When an absolute is desired, both counts are reported. In the case of a simple arch there is no triradius, therefore, no ridge count.

The normal mean ridge count of 10 digits: MALES   145
FEMALES   126

CLASSIFICATION OF SOLE PRINTS

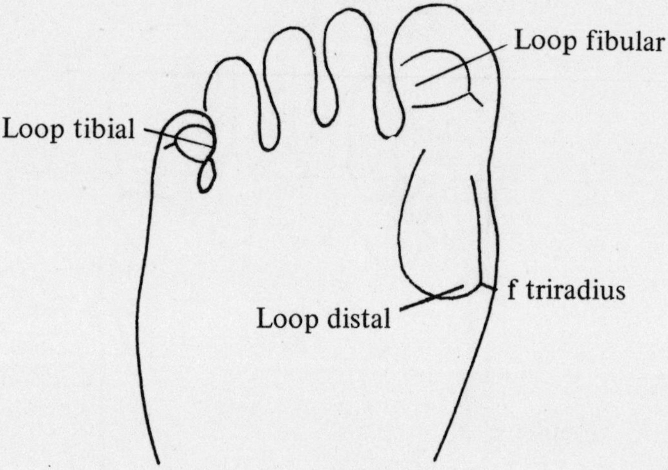

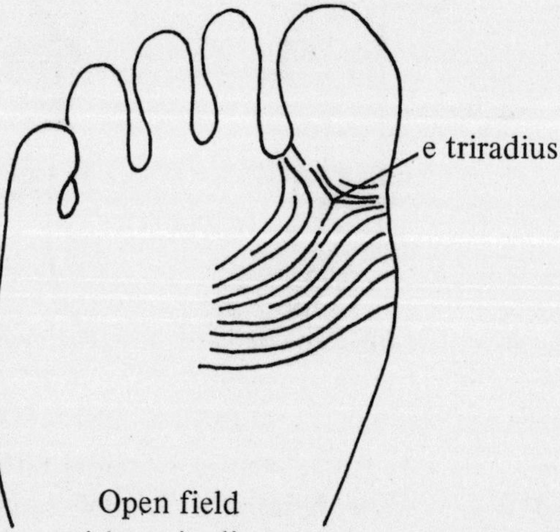

Open field
with e triradius

CLASSIFICATION OF SOLE PRINTS (Continued)

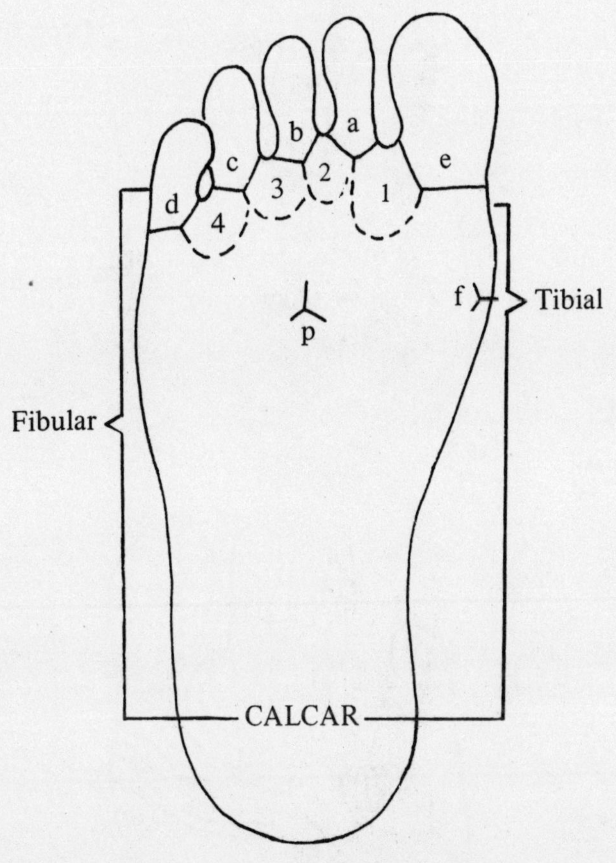

1, 2, 3, 4 = Interdigital areas
e, a, b, c, d = Digital triradii
f, p = Hallucal triradii

GRAPHIC ILLUSTRATION OF HAND PRINT

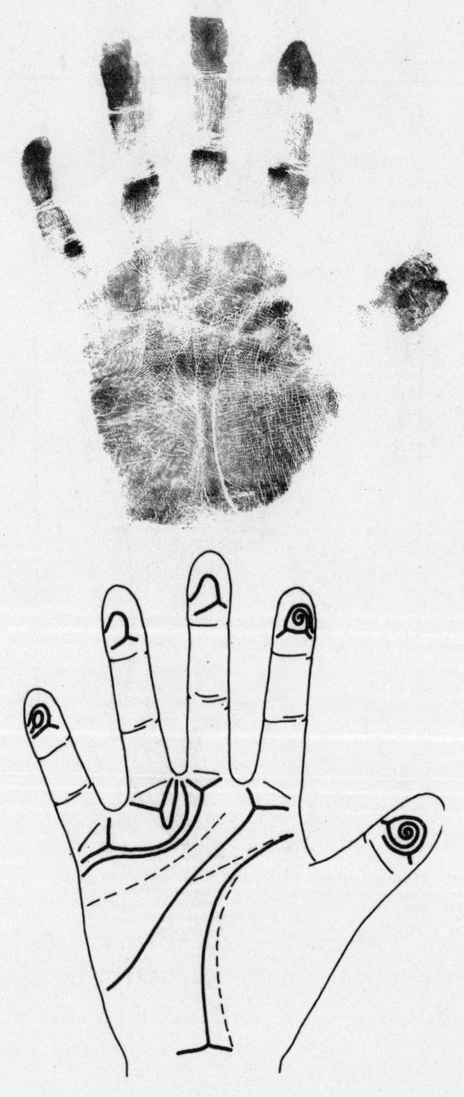

GRAPHIC ILLUSTRATION OF FOOT PRINT

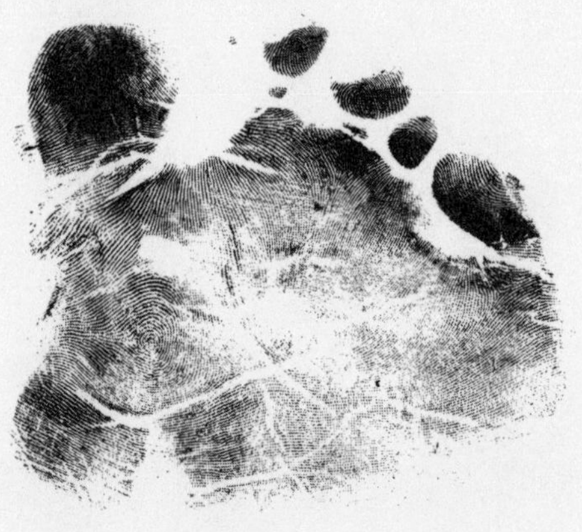

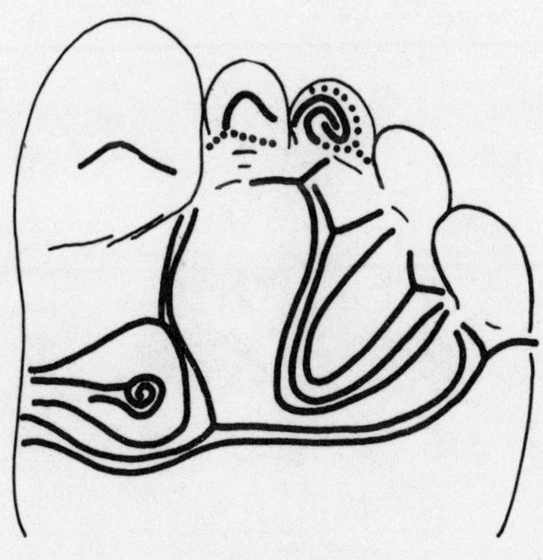

4

Dermatoglyphs in Autosomal Chromosome Aberrations

DOWN'S SYNDROME (MONGOLISM)

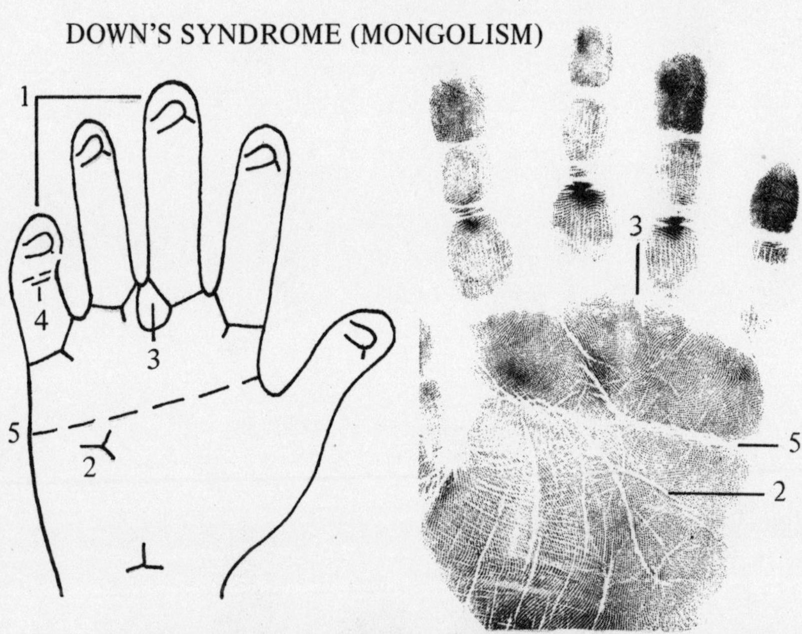

1. 10 ulnar loops in more than 80% (occurs in about 60% of normals). Radial loops on digits 4 and 5 occurs more frequently in mongols. In normals a radial loop is present on digit 2.

2. *atd* angle increased, greater than 57%. (Axial triradius at *t''*.)

3. Pattern in third interdigital space. (Occurs in 95.5% mongols and 40.8% normal.)

4. Single crease on little finger. (20-30% of mongols.)

5. Simian line. (Occurs in 58% of mongols, less than 5% of normal.)

DOWN'S SYNDROME (Continued)

6.   Tibial arch. Most useful pattern when present. (Occurs in 45% of mongols either left or right foot. In normals less than 0.5%.)

7.   Distal loop. Fourth interdigital area of foot. (Occurs twice as often in mongols as in non-mongols.)

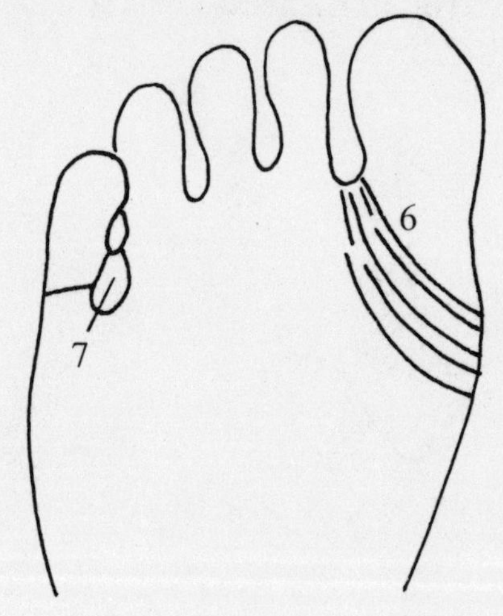

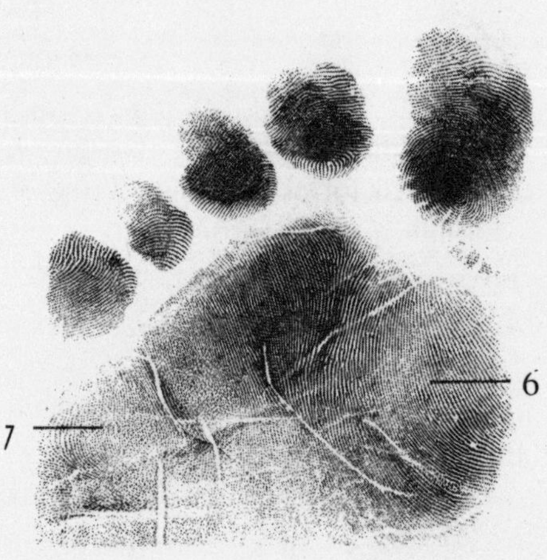

VARIANT OF DOWN'S SYNDROME

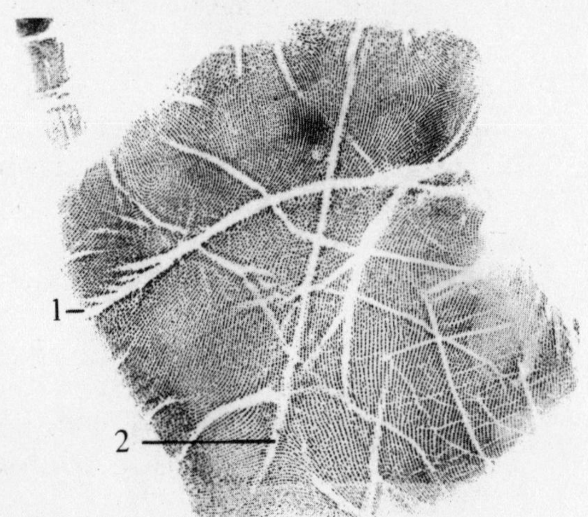

1. Simian Crease.
2. t' triradius.
3. 4th interdigital distal loop.
4. Small distal loop (ridge count under 20).

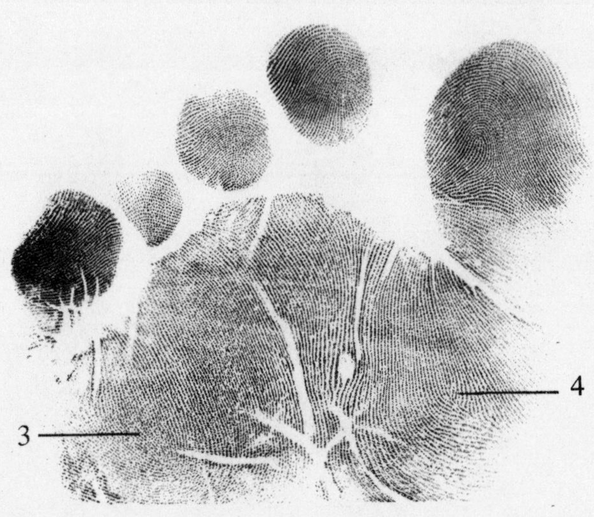

TRISOMY D
(Extra Chromosome in 13-15 Group)

1. *atd* angle increased. (77% have marked increases in angle. Mean sum of both *atd* angles varies between 186-196 degrees with 93-98 degrees for normal.)

2. Radial loops on fourth and fifth digits. (Rare in general population.)

3. Increased arches. (19% of digits show arches as opposed 5% of normal.)

4. Patterns in thenar and first interdigital area. (Occur in 50% of hands.)

5. Arch fibular (S pattern) with an *f* triradius and elongated fibular loop related to *d* triradius.

6. Tibial loop.

TRISOMY D (Continued)

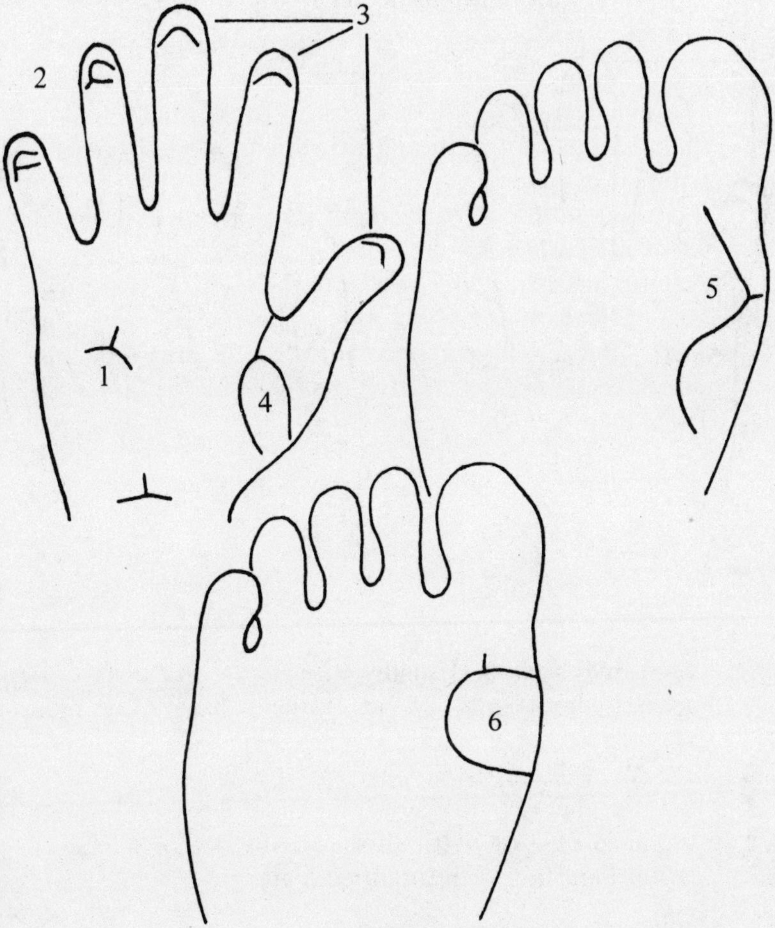

TRISOMY E
(Extra Chromosome in 17-18 Group)

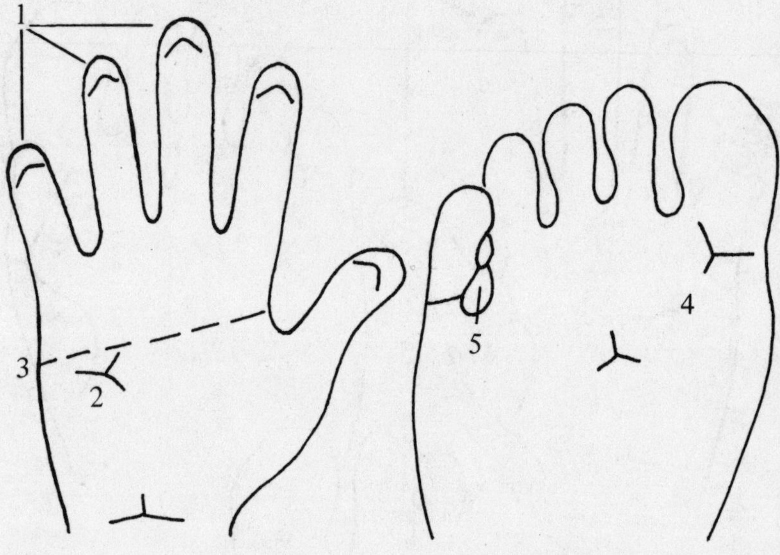

1. Increased arches. (Usually 6 or more, some have 10 arches; about only 2% of normals have 6 or more arches.)
2. *atd* angle increased. (Axial triradius at *t''*.)
3. Simian line.
4. Presence of *e* or *p* triradius and absence of *f* in soles.
5. Distal loop in fourth interdigital area.

CAT CRY SYNDROME
(Deletion of Chromosome #5)

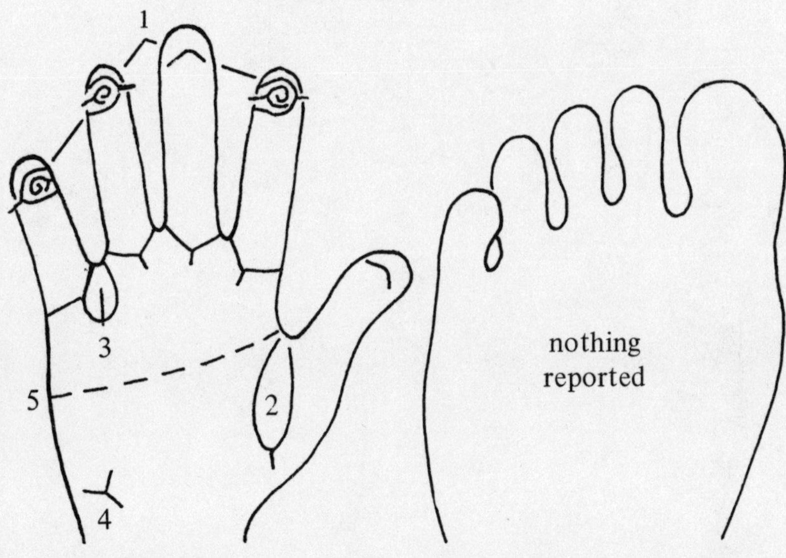

nothing reported

1. Increased whorls and arches.
2. Thenar pattern. (Occurs in 42% as opposed 12.5% normal.)
3. Fourth interdigital loop.
4. *atd* angle increased. (Axial triradius at *t'*.)
5. Simian line.

Dermatoglyphs in Sex Chromosome Aberrations

TURNER'S SYNDROME
(XO Chromosome Compliment)

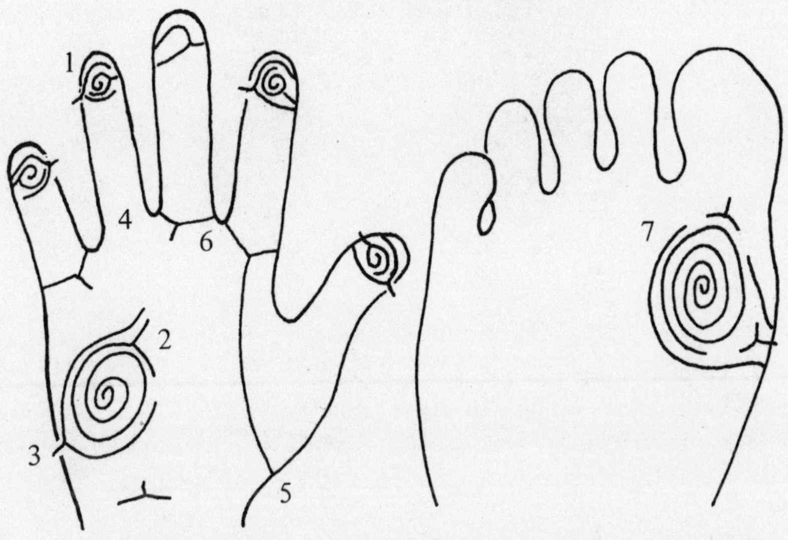

1. Increased whorls and large loops. (Ridge count increased: 166-178. General population of females 126.)
2. *atd* angle increased. (Axial triradius at t''.)
3. Large hypothenar pattern. (Occurs in 66% of patients, 12% normal.)
4. Missing *c* triradius.
5. *A* line exiting in the thenar area.
6. Increased *ab* ridge count.
7. Large whorls and distal loops are frequent. *p* triradius is missing.

VARIANT OF TURNER'S SYNDROME

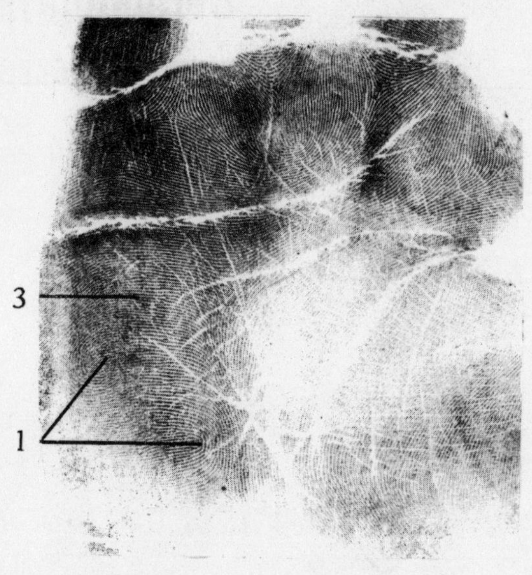

1. Large S loop.
2. Large ulnar loops . In digits (not shown).
3. *t''* triradius.

KLINEFELTER'S SYNDROME
(XXY Chromosome Compliment)

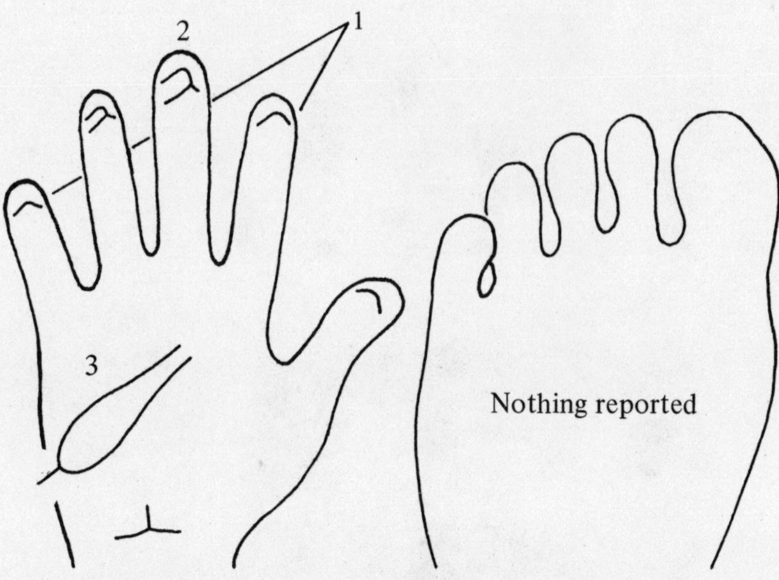

1. Increased arches.
2. Mean total ridge count reduced to 114. (Normal male 145.)
3. Hypothenar pattern. (Occurs in 36% as opposed 25% normal.)

VARIANT OF KLINEFELTER'S SYNDROME

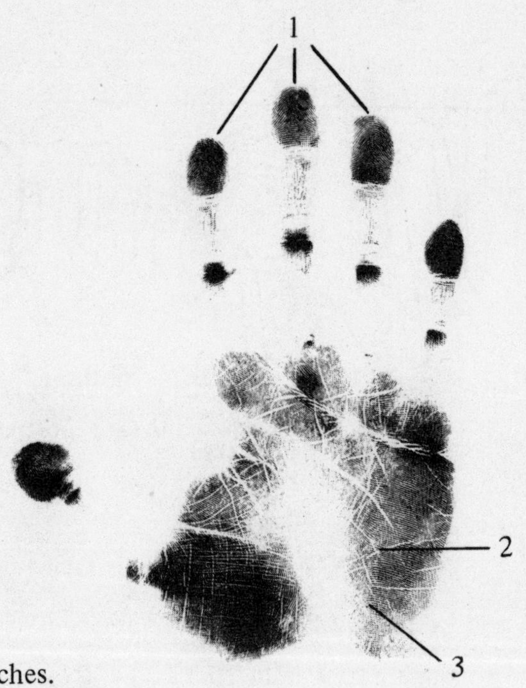

1. Arches.
2. *t'* triradius.
3. Arch carpal.

XYY SYNDROME

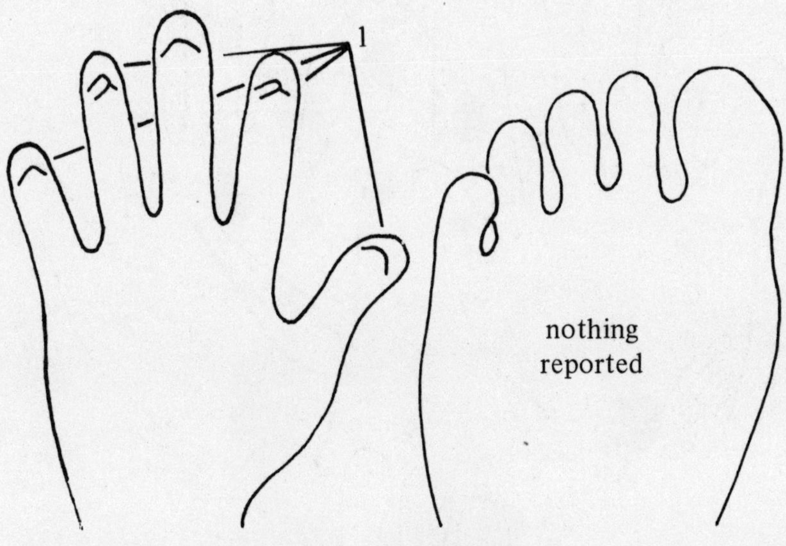

1. Increased arches.
2. Decrease of total ridge count: 109-114.

XXYY SYNDROME

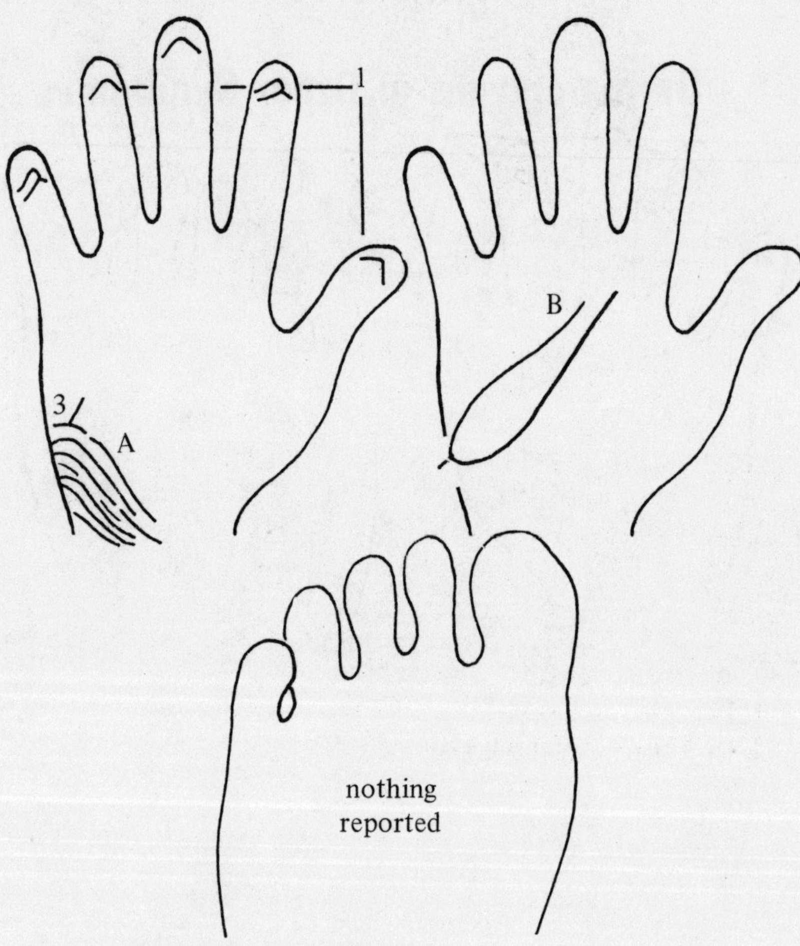

1.   Increased arches (occurs in 17%).
2.   Mean ridge count reduced to 90-106.
3.   *atd* angle increased. Axial triradius associated with either arch-carpal (A) or loop-radial (B) hypothenar pattern.
4.   Sole dermatoglyphs not helpful.

6

Dermatoglyphs in Other Syndromes

de LANGE SYNDROME

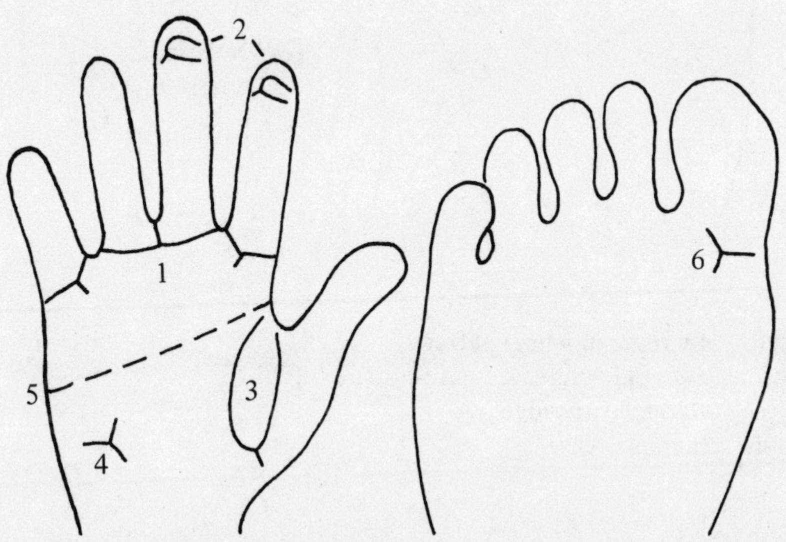

1. Interdigital triradius—usually in the third interspace.
2. Radial loops found on second and third digits.
3. Large loop in the thenar area.
4. *atd* angle increased. (Axial triradius at *t'*.)
5. Simian crease.
6. Open field with an *e* triradius.

PRENATAL RUBELLA SYNDROME

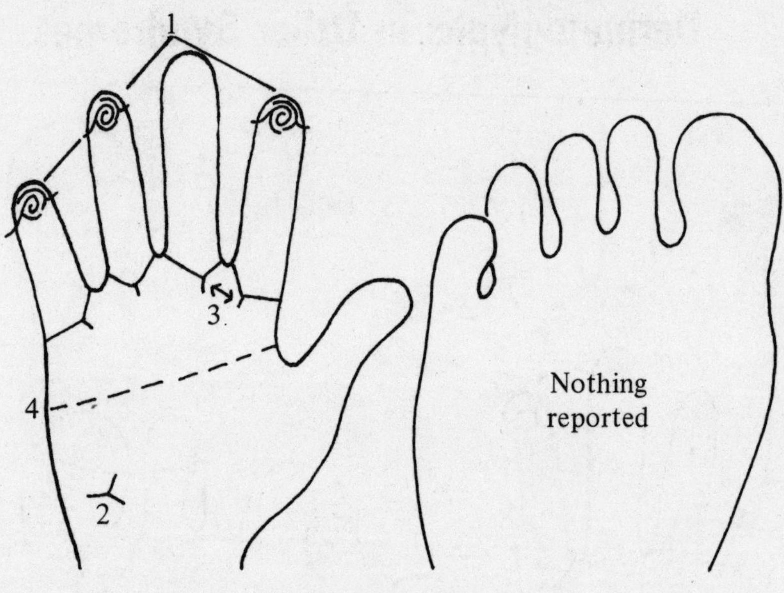

1. Increase in whorl pattern.
2. *atd* angle increased. (Axial triradius at *t'*.)
3. Reduced *ab* ridge count.
4. Simian crease.

RUBINSTEIN SYNDROME
Broad Toes and Thumb Syndrome

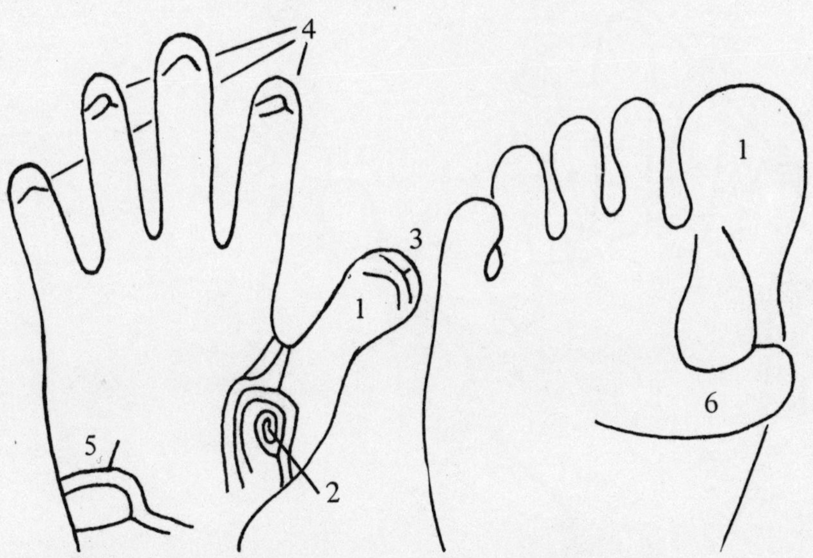

1.   Broad big toes and thumbs.
2.   Large and complex thenar pattern.
3.   Extra triradius tip of thumb or big toe.
4.   Reduced total ridge count.
5.   Ulnar loop in the hypothenar area associated with an increased *atd* angle. (Axial triradius at *t'*.)
6.   Distal loop with the *f* triradius displaced toward tibial border of foot and associated with a loop opening toward the fibular border.

7

Syndromes with Indefinite Dermatoglyphic Findings

HYPERCALCEMIA

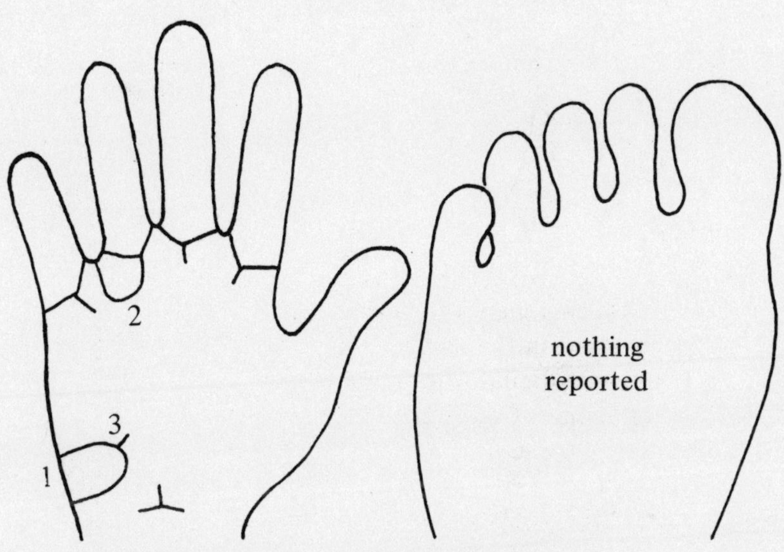

1. Small ulnar loop in hypothenar area.
2. Distal loop in fourth interspace.
3. Increased *atd* angle.

CEREBRAL GIGANTISM

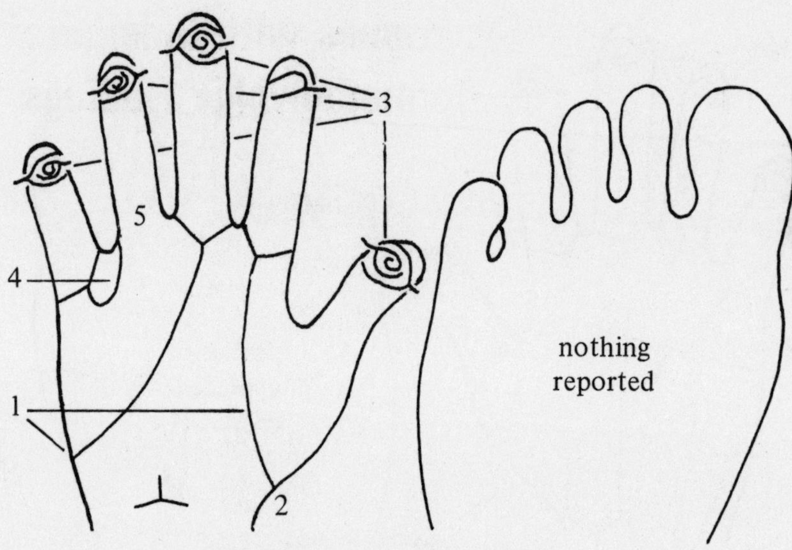

1. Vertical alignment of main lines.
2. *A* line exits in the thenar area.
3. Increase in digital whorls and loops.
4. Distal loop in fourth interspace.
5. Missing *c* triradius.

SMITH-LEMLI-OPITZ SYNDROME

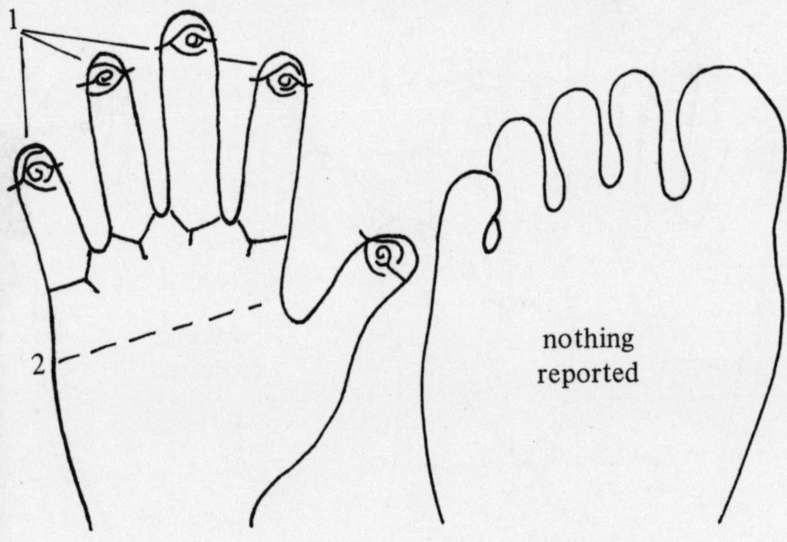

1. Increased whorls producing a high ridge count.
2. Simian crease.

PRADER-WILLI SYNDROME

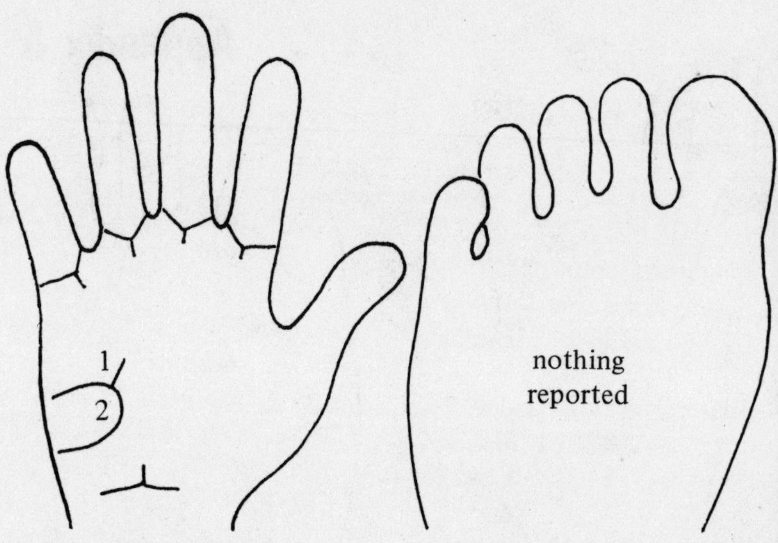

1. *atd* angle greater than 57°.
2. Hypothenar loop.

Appendix A

Normal Values

Total ridge count (Holt, 1955):
     145   - Males
     126   - Females

Bilateral *ab* ridge count (Pons, 1964):
     82   - Males
     84   - Females

Bilateral *atd* angle (Penrose):

92.5	Males	(ages 0-4)
97.5	Females	
88.5	Males	(ages 5-14)
89.8	Females	
85.0	Males	(ages 15-)
85.9	Females	

Finger patterns (Holt, English controls):

Whorls	26.1%
Ulnar loops	63.5%
Radial loops	5.4%
Arches	5.0%

HAND AND FOOT OUTLINES

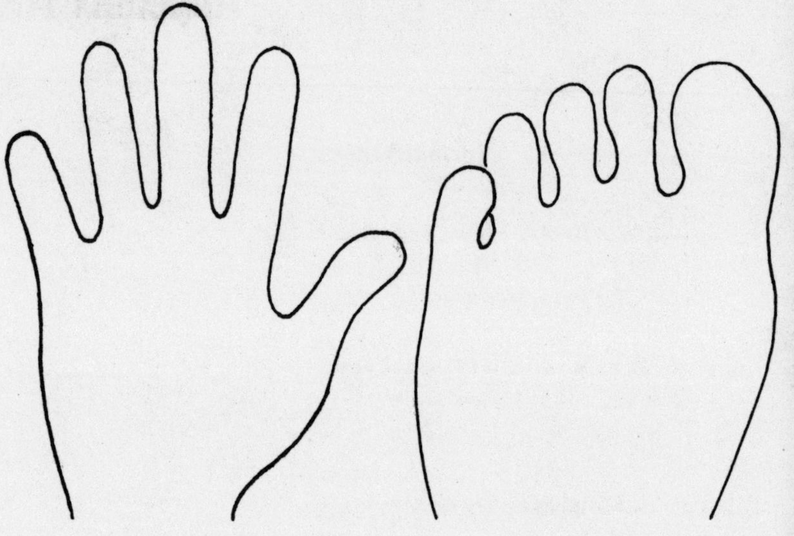

Appendix B

Materials

\# 800 - Resensitizing fluid
\# 240 - Hand applicator
Palm print paper (7 1/2" x 8 1/2")
   Faurot, Inc.
   299 Broadway
   New York, N.Y. 10007

\# 5802 - Glossy paper (4" x 6 1/2")
Disposable footprinter
Graphite - dry footprinter
   Hollister, Inc.
   211 East Chicago Avenue
   Chicago, Ill. 60611

Flash magnifier
   Selsi Company
   Japan

Fingerprint ink
   Searche Laboratories, Inc.
   Morristown, N.J. 07960

Bibliography

Achs, R.; Harper, R.; and Siegel, M.: Unusual Dermato-glyphic Finding Associated with Rubella Embryopathy, *New Eng J Med* 274 (Jan) 1966.

Alter, M.: Dermatoglyphic Analysis as a Diagnostic Tool, *Med* 46: 1-12, 1966.

Bartlett, D. J., et al: Chromosomes of Male Patients in a Security Prison, *Nat* 219 (July 27) 1968.

Berg, J. M., et al: Partial Deletion of Short Arm of a Chromosome of the 4-5 Group (Denver) in an Adult Male, *J Ment Def Res* 9 (Dec. pt 4) 1965.

Borgaonkar, D. S., et al: The YY Syndrome, *Lancet* 2:461-162, 1968.

Cummins, H., and Mildo, D.: *Finger Prints, Palms and Soles,* Philadelphia: Blackinston Co., 1943.

Ford Walker, N.: The Use of Dermal Configurations in the Diagnosis of Mongolism, *J Ped* 50:19-26, 1957.

Galton, F.: *Finger Prints,* London: MacMillan, 1892.

Holt, S. B.: *The Genetics of Dermal Ridges,* Springfield, Ill.: Charles C. Thomas, Publisher, 1968.

Hunter, H.: Finger and Palm Prints in Chromatin-positive Males, *J Md Genet* 5:112, 1968.

Penrose, L. S.: The Distal Triradius "t" on the Hands of Parents and Sibs of Mongol Imbeciles, *Ann Hum Genet* (London) 19:10-38, 1954.

Penrose, L. S.: Memorandum on Dermatoglyphic Nomen-clature, *Bir Def* 4, No. 3 (June) 1968.

Penrose, L. S., and Smith, G. F.: *Down's Anomaly,* Boston: Little, Brown and Co., 1966.

Pons, J.: Quantitative Genetics of Palmar Dermatoglyphics, *Amer J Hum Genet* 11:252, 1959.

Smith, G. F.: Dermatoglyphic Patterns on the Fourth Inter-digital Area of the Sole in Down's Syndrome, *J Ment Def Res* 8 (Dec. pt 2) 1964.

Smith, G. F.: A Study of the Dermatoglyphs in the deLange Syndrome, *J Ment Def Res* 10 (Dec. pt 4) 1966.

Smith, G. F.; Ridler, M. A. C.; and Bat-Miriam, M.: Dermal Patterns on the Fingers and Toes in Mongolism, *J Ment Def Res* 10 (June, pt 2) 1966.

Telfer, M. A., et al: Incidence of Gross Chromosomal Errors Among Tall Criminal American Men, *Science* 159:1249-1250.

Uchida, I. A.; Patau, K.; and Smith, D. W.: The Dermal Pattern of the New Autosomal Trisomy Syndromes, *Amer J Dis Child* 102:588, 1961.

Warburton, D., and Miller, O. J.: Dermatoglyphic Features of Patients with a Partial Short Arm Deletion of a B-group Chromosome, *Ann Hum Genet* (London) 31:189, 1967.